50 Juice Recipes to Lower Your Blood Pressure:

An Easy Way to Reduce High Blood Pressure

By

Joseph Correa

Certified Sports Nutritionist

COPYRIGHT

© 2016 Finibi Inc

All rights reserved

Reproduction or translation of any part of this work beyond that permitted by section 107 or 108 of the 1976 United States Copyright Act without the permission of the copyright owner is unlawful.

This publication is designed to provide accurate and authoritative information in regard to the subject matter covered. It is sold with the understanding that neither the author nor the publisher is engaged in rendering medical advice. If medical advice or assistance is needed, consult with a doctor. This book is considered a guide and should not be used in any way detrimental to your health. Consult with a physician before starting this nutritional plan to make sure it's right for you.

ACKNOWLEDGEMENTS

The realization and success of this book could not have been possible without the motivation and support of my entire family.

50 Juice Recipes to Lower Your Blood Pressure: An Easy Way to Reduce High Blood Pressure

By

Joseph Correa

Certified Sports Nutritionist

CONTENTS

Copyright

Acknowledgements

About The Author

Introduction

50 Juice Recipes to Lower Your Blood Pressure: An Easy Way to Reduce High Blood Pressure

Other Great Titles by This Author

ABOUT THE AUTHOR

As a certified sports nutritionist, I honestly believe in the positive effects that proper nutrition can have over the body and mind. My knowledge and experience has helped me live healthier throughout the years and which I have shared with family and friends. The more you know about eating and drinking healthier, the sooner you will want to change your life and eating habits.

Nutrition is a key part in the process of being healthy and living longer so get started today.

INTRODUCTION

50 Juice Recipes to Lower Your Blood Pressure will help you to control your blood pressure better naturally and fast. Hypertension is a serious health problem that should be addressed with exercise and proper nutrition. These are not to replace meals but should complement your normal day to day meals.

Being too busy to eat right can sometimes become a problem and that's why this book will save you time and help nourish your body to achieve the goals you want.

This book will help you to:

-Lower Your High Blood Pressure

-Reduce Fat.

-Cleanse Your Blood Stream.

-Have more energy.

-Naturally accelerate Your Metabolism to become thinner.

-Improve your digestive system.

Joseph Correa is a certified sports nutritionist and a professional athlete.

50 JUICE RECIPES TO LOWER YOUR BLOOD PRESSURE

1. Surprise Sunrise

This juice recipe is a problem solver when it comes to issues with high blood pressure. It's rich in vitamins and minerals that will turn your body into a healthy energy factory.

Benefits:

Celery is well known for having a high calcium content. Celery helps controlling high blood pressure. Pears have anti-oxidants which help prevent high blood pressure.

Ingredients:

- Apples - 2 medium 360g
- Carrots - 2 medium 122g
- Celery - 3 stalk, large 190g
- Lemons (peeled) - 2 fruit 165g

- Pears - 2 medium 356g

How to prepare:

- **Wash all the ingredients thoroughly.**
- **Juice them well and enjoy this fresh drink right away.**

Total calories: 381

Vitamins: Vitamin A 785ug, Vitamin C 187mg, Calcium 130mg

Minerals: Sodium 221mg, Potassium 2454mg

Sugars 55g

2. Light Cream

The best way to keep you relaxed and full of energy during the day is to start with a natural juice. Here is a great recipe that will do more than that, check it out.

Benefits:

Certain protein compounds that you find only in spinach are great to lower high blood pressure. Bell pepper is known to reduce cholesterol and high blood pressure.

Ingredients:

- Cucumber - 1/2 cucumber 150g
- Parsley - 2 handful 80g
- Pepper - 1/2 medium 59g
- Spinach - 1 cup 30g
- Tomatoes - 3 medium whole 350g
- Cabbage (red) - 1 leaf 22g

How to prepare:

- **Wash all the ingredients thoroughly.**

- **Juice them well and enjoy this fresh drink right away.**

Total calories: 115

Vitamins: Vitamin A 205ug, Vitamin C 97mg, Calcium 221mg

Minerals: Sodium 212mg, Potassium 1755mg

Sugars 13g

3. Mind Lifting

A variety of fruits and vegetables make this a great to have a healthy body. That's why this recipe is a powerful and healthy one, and you should try it in the morning.

Benefits:

A recent study has shown that foods high in potassium lower blood pressure as well. Oranges are a great source of vitamin C.

Ingredients:

- Cucumber - 1 cucumber 300g
- Oranges - 2 fruit 260g
- Pineapple - 1/4 fruit 226.25g
- Spinach - 5 handful 125g
- Banana – 1 medium 90g

How to prepare:

- **Wash all the ingredients thoroughly.**
- **Juice them well and enjoy this fresh drink right away.**

Total calories: 184

Vitamins: Vitamin A 421ug, Vitamin C 154mg, Calcium 202mg

Minerals: Sodium 71mg, Potassium 1322mg

Sugars 30g

4. HT Juice

When you want a healthy body and mind you should add different juice recipes that include leafy vegetables and mixing them with better tasting ingredients to improve the flavor of the drink.

Benefits:

Lime juice is helpful for people that suffer heart problems because it contains potassium. It also helps to control blood pressure, and reduces mental stress.

Ingredients:

- Apples - 2 medium 364g
- Kale - 5 leaf 175g
- Lime - 1/2 fruit 32g
- Orange - 150g
- Carrots -1 large 70g

How to prepare:

- **Wash all the ingredients thoroughly.**

- **Juice them well and enjoy this fresh drink right away.**

Total calories: 160

Vitamins: Vitamin A 300ug, Vitamin C 191mg, Calcium 109mg

Minerals: Sodium 103mg, Potassium 1437mg

Sugars 43g

5. Big A

You can always use a new juice recipe that contains all essential minerals and vitamins that will lead your body in the end to a healthier one. This is another great morning drink.

Benefits:

Pectin in apples lowers cholesterol levels and can also help lower blood pressure. Pear juice has an anti-inflammatory effect and is a very good nutrient provider.

Ingredients:

- Apples - 2 medium 360g
- Orange (peeled) - 1 fruit 130g
- Pears - 2 medium 356g
- Sweet Potato - 130g
- Lime ½ - 33g

How to prepare:

- **Wash all the ingredients thoroughly.**

- **Juice them well and enjoy this fresh drink right away.**

Total calories: 307

Vitamins: Vitamin A 610ug, Vitamin C 61mg, Calcium 123mg

Minerals: Sodium 120mg, Potassium 1221mg

Sugars 60g

6. Sweet Day

This juice recipe is a great one if you want a positive change in your heart. If you have had heart problems in the past try this drink and see what it may do for you.

Benefits:

Beets have medicinal properties, they help normalize blood pressure, and they also are high in carbohydrates, a great source of instant energy.

Ingredients:

- Beet Root (golden) - 1 beet 80g
- Carrots - 3 large 215g
- Cucumber - 1/2 cucumber 150g
- Ginger Root - 1/2 thumb 12g
- Lime- ½ 33g

How to prepare:

- **Wash all the ingredients thoroughly.**
- **Juice them well and enjoy this fresh drink right away.**

Total calories: 137

Vitamins: Vitamin A 1104ug, Vitamin C 19mg, Calcium 143mg

Minerals: Sodium 265mg, Potassium 1391mg

Sugars 22g

7. Green God

You should try this juice recipe at lunch because it's very rich in nutrients that will be better absorbed during that time of the day and be easier for you to digest.

Benefits:

Cucumber is an essential component of healthy connective tissue, and it also helps lower blood pressure.

Ingredients:

- Celery - 4 stalk, large 255g
- Cucumber - 1 cucumber 300g
- Ginger Root - 1 thumb 24g
- Lemon - 1/2 fruit 42g

How to prepare:

- **Wash all the ingredients thoroughly.**
- **Juice them well and enjoy this fresh drink right away.**

Total calories: 183

Vitamins: Vitamin A 764ug, Vitamin C 171mg, Calcium 312mg

Minerals: Sodium 195mg, Potassium 1872mg

Sugars 30g

8. Healing Mix

Here is another great juice recipe that will help you improve your health and the way you feel. If the combination of lemon and orange is too strong for you, simply eliminate one of the two but if you can drink them together it will be better.

Benefits:

Lemon juice reduces depression and controls high blood pressure, and consuming vitamin C helps to lower the incidence of peptic ulcers.

Ingredients:

- Celery - 4 stalk, large 255g
- Lemon (with rind) - 1/2 fruit 28g
- Orange (peeled) - 1 large 180g
- Spinach - 5 handful 125g

How to prepare:

- **Wash all the ingredients thoroughly.**

- **Juice them well and enjoy this fresh drink right away.**

Total calories: 202

Vitamins: Vitamin A 250ug, Vitamin C 87mg, Calcium 211mg

Minerals: Sodium 211mg, Potassium 1501mg

Sugars 40g

9. GROWL Juice

Juice recipes are a fast way to keep up with a modern lifestyle for individuals that are looking to have a healthy body. This is a great recipe to lower blood pressure and strengthen your heart.

Benefits:

Ginger might have a role in lowering cholesterol and also helps lower high blood pressure. The extract from apple skin may lower risk of liver cancer so it would be better if you wash well and include the skin when juicing.

Ingredients:

- Apples - 2 medium 365g
- Celery - 3 stalk, large 192g
- Cucumber - 1 cucumber 300g
- Lime (with rind) - 1 fruit 65g
- Parsley - 1 bunch 150g

How to prepare:

- **Wash all the ingredients thoroughly.**

- **Juice them well and enjoy this fresh drink right away.**

Total calories: 202

Vitamins: Vitamin A 590ug, Vitamin C 156mg, Calcium 281mg

Minerals: Sodium 197mg, Potassium 1789mg

Sugars 28g

10. All Star Juice

Start your day strong with this great mix of fruits and delicious vegetables. These ingredients are perfect for you because they are rich in nutrients and vitamins.

Benefits:

Pears contain anti-carcinogen glutathione that helps prevent blood pressure. Carrots are rich in beta-carotene and they also may reduce high blood pressure.

Ingredients:

- Carrots - 4 medium 220g
- Cucumber - 1 cucumber 300g
- Lemon - 1 fruit 58g
- Pear - 1 medium 178g
- Celery - 1 stalk, large 62g

How to prepare:

- **Wash all the ingredients thoroughly.**
- **Juice them well and enjoy this fresh drink right away.**

Total calories: 210

Vitamins: Vitamin A 1044ug, Vitamin C 40mg, Calcium 139mg

Minerals: Sodium 149mg, Potassium 1451mg

Sugars 32g

11. Junior Juice

When each second is precious and you feel like you are running out of time to get healthier, you should not neglect your body, that is why this awesome juice recipe will do wonders for you and your body in a very short period of time.

Benefits:

Celery is great for lowering high blood pressure and it's a great source of nutrients.

Ingredients:

- Celery - 3 stalk, large 190g
- Cucumber - 1/2 cucumber 150g
- Ginger Root - 1/2 thumb 12g
- Kale - 2 leaf 70g
- Banana - 1 medium 90g

How to prepare:

- **Wash all the ingredients thoroughly.**

- **Juice them well and enjoy this fresh drink right away.**

Total calories: 200

Vitamins: Vitamin A 503ug, Vitamin C 176mg, Calcium 276mg

Minerals: Sodium 133mg, Potassium 1569mg

Sugars 45g

12. Mr. Heart Healthy Mix

Make sure you start your day with this heart healthy mix with a great flavor thanks to the banana and apple combination.

Benefits:

Bananas play an important role in reducing blood pressure. Apples lower cholesterol and also increase bone density.

Ingredients:

- Carrots - 4 medium 242g
- Celery - 3 stalk, large 190g
- Ginger Root - 1/2 thumb 11g
- Banana – 1 medium 90g
- Apple – 1 medium 180g

How to prepare:

- **Wash all the ingredients thoroughly.**
- **Juice them well and enjoy this fresh drink right away.**

Total calories: 233

Vitamins: Vitamin A 1312ug, Vitamin C 27mg, Calcium 143mg

Minerals: Sodium 310mg, Potassium 1670mg

Sugars 44g

13. Sunny Start Breakfast Drink

Here is a great juice recipe that you can start your day with. It will keep your energy levels high during the entire day and will also be an excellent source of vitamins, so check it out.

Benefits:

Tomatoes have been known to be excellent for your heart and may lower their blood pressure. They are also a great source of vitamin C.

Ingredients:

- Apples (green) - 1 medium 180g
- Cucumber - 1 cucumber 300g
- Grapes (green) - 15 grape 90g
- Spinach - 2 cup 60g
- Tomato - 1 medium whole 121g

How to prepare:

- **Wash all the ingredients thoroughly.**

- **Juice them well and enjoy this fresh drink right away.**

Total calories: 179

Vitamins: Vitamin A 540ug, Vitamin C 59mg, Calcium 144mg

Minerals: Sodium 112mg, Potassium 1448mg

Sugars 31g

14. Beet Rain Delay

If you're ready to start a healthy habit, juicing is a wonderful idea. The sweet potato in this drink will give it a new tasteful flavor you will enjoy.

Benefits:

Medical studies have shown that including beets in your diet help protect your body against heart disease. They also help regenerate red blood cells and supply fresh oxygen to the body.

Ingredients:

- Apple - 1 medium 180g
- Beet Root - 1 beet 170g
- Lemon - 1/2 fruit 42g
- Oranges (peeled) - 2 fruit 262g
- Sweet Potato - 1 130g

How to prepare:

- **Wash all the ingredients thoroughly.**

- **Juice them well and enjoy this fresh drink right away.**

Total calories: 245

Vitamins: Vitamin A 450ug, Vitamin C 87mg, Calcium 137mg

Minerals: Sodium 227mg, Potassium 1894mg

Sugars 34g

15. Rainbow Parade

The world of science is still discovering new things about how important vegetables and fruits are to our lives. Here is a great example of a juice recipe that will make you want to add them to your everyday meals.

Benefits:

A recent study has shown that foods rich in magnesium and fiber help the body drop blood pressure to healthier levels. Spinach is a great blood builder and regenerates red cells.

Ingredients:

- Celery - 4 stalk, medium 160g
- Cucumber - 1/2 cucumber 150g
- Grapes - 2 cup 180g
- Spinach - 4 cup 120g

How to prepare:

- **Wash all the ingredients thoroughly.**

- **Juice them well and enjoy this fresh drink right away.**

Total calories: 219

Vitamins: Vitamin A 322ug, Vitamin C 37mg, Calcium 179mg

Minerals: Sodium 144mg, Potassium 1671mg

Sugars 38g

16. Smiling Pineapple Mix

Here is another recipe that you should try. Share it with your family because it's really an amazing one if you like pineapple.

Benefits:

Drinking lemon juice is great for the heart and it also helps controls high blood pressure. A carrot a day reduces stroke risk by about 66 percent.

Ingredients:

- Carrots - 3 medium 180g
- Lemon - 1/2 fruit 40g
- Pineapple - 1/4 fruit 225g
- Spinach - 2 handful 50g

How to prepare:

- **Wash all the ingredients thoroughly.**
- **Juice them well and enjoy this fresh drink right away.**

Total calories: 202

Vitamins: Vitamin A 975ug, Vitamin C 150mg, Calcium 165mg

Minerals: Sodium 210mg, Potassium 1410mg

Sugars 37g

17. Cranberry Delight Juice

This juice recipe is unusual with a variety of ingredients you won't normally find anywhere so give it a try and notice the spectacular results you'll have.

Benefits:

Oranges being high in vitamin C can help stimulate white cells to fight different infections, and a recent study has linked them to lower blood pressure.

Ingredients:

- Cranberries - 3 cup, 300g
- Ginger Root - 2 thumb 45g
- Limes (with rind) - 2 fruit 134g
- Banana – 1 medium 90g

How to prepare:

- **Wash all the ingredients thoroughly.**
- **Juice them well and enjoy this fresh drink right away.**

Total calories: 285

Vitamins: Vitamin A 145ug, Vitamin C 219mg, Calcium 172mg

Minerals: Sodium 7mg, Potassium 1128mg

Sugars 48g

18. Kale Vow

Kale is full of necessary vitamins and minerals that will help your body reduce high blood pressure and make you feel much better during the day. Add some more leaves if you don't mind the added flavor as it will only make more nutritious.

Benefits:

Kale contains different compounds that lower high blood pressure and recent studies shown that lemons help in reducing cholesterol.

Ingredients:

- Apples - 2 medium 320g
- Kale - 2 leaf (8-12") 70g
- Lemon (peeled) - 1 fruit 58g
- Tomato - 1 medium whole 120g

How to prepare:

- **Wash all the ingredients thoroughly.**

- **Juice them well and enjoy this fresh drink right away.**

Total calories: 275

Vitamins: Vitamin A 434ug, Vitamin C 91mg, Calcium 201mg

Minerals: Sodium 190mg, Potassium 1448mg

Sugars 45g

19. Carroty Lime Max

This is a great juice to serve after or during a big meal. The combination of lime and pepper give it a kick in flavor but the banana makes it sweet tasting. If you feel it is still too strong in flavor simply add half a banana more.

Benefits:

Regular consumption of carrots reduces cholesterol levels and to prevent heart related problems. They also help cleanse the liver.

Ingredients:

- Carrots - 2 large 170g
- Celery - 2 stalk, large 128g
- Lime - 1/2 fruit 32g
- Pepper - 1 pepper 14g
- Spinach - 2 cup 60g
- Banana – 1 medium 90g

How to prepare:

- **Wash all the ingredients thoroughly.**

- **Juice them well and enjoy this fresh drink right away.**

Total calories: 110

Vitamins: Vitamin A 875ug, Vitamin C 32mg, Calcium 127mg

Minerals: Sodium 255mg, Potassium 1329mg

Sugars 15g

20. Cucumber High

If having a healthy body is your goal you have to try this juice recipe. You can lower the amount of onion if you don't like the flavor but it would be recommended you keep it in because of the health benefits.

Benefits:

Parsley has been shown to function as antioxidant and help maintain a healthy level of blood pressure. Tomato juice is an excellent source of vitamin C, calcium and phosphorous.

Ingredients:

- Cucumber - 1 cucumber 300g
- Lemon - 1 fruit 55g
- Onion - 15g
- Parsley - 1 handful 40g
- Tomatoes - 2 small whole 180g

How to prepare:

- **Wash all the ingredients thoroughly.**

- **Juice them well and enjoy this fresh drink right away.**

Total calories: 79

Vitamins: Vitamin A 255ug, Vitamin C 105mg, Calcium 98mg

Minerals: Sodium 30mg, Potassium 1077mg

Sugars 10g

21. Broc Mix

Let's see if this delicious juice recipe is what you are looking for. One of the great things about juice recipes is that they don't take much time to prepare and the results are outstanding.

Benefits:

Broccoli helps in proper functioning of insulin and regulates blood sugar, thereby regulating blood pressure also.

Ingredients:

- Apple - 1 medium 180g
- Broccoli - 1 stalk 150g
- Carrots - 2 large 110g
- Celery - 3 stalk, large 190g
- Olive Oil - 1 tablespoon 13.5g

How to prepare:

- **Wash all the ingredients thoroughly.**

- **Juice them well and enjoy this fresh drink right away.**

Total calories: 224

Vitamins: Vitamin A 1003ug, Vitamin C 110mg, Calcium 196mg

Minerals: Sodium 215mg, Potassium 1335mg

Sugars 19g

22. Blueberry Surprise Mix

Blueberries taste great and are wonderful anti-oxidants. Mixing these ingredients will give you a great juice to drink at any time of the day not just the morning.

Benefits:

Vitamins make our system function properly and are found in abundance in blueberries. Blueberries also help to maintain a strong immune system.

Ingredients:

- Apple - 1 medium 180g
- Blueberry - 1 cup 140g
- Broccoli - 1 stalk 151g
- Tomato - 1 medium whole 120g

How to prepare:

- **Wash all the ingredients thoroughly.**
- **Juice them well and enjoy this fresh drink right away.**

Total calories: 203

Vitamins: Vitamin A 784ug, Vitamin C 102mg, Calcium 115mg

Minerals: Sodium 188mg, Potassium 1431mg

Sugars 39g

23. Fit Ginger Juice

Here is another great juice recipe that you can enjoy at any moment of the day, just make sure you prepare it with 30 minutes before any big meal.

Benefits:

Pectin in carrots lowers the serum cholesterol levels and is also rich in vitamin A which is good for improving eyesight.

Ingredients:

- Carrots - 2 medium 120g
- Ginger Root - 1/2 12g
- Lemon - 1 fruit 50g
- Spinach - 2 handful 50g

How to prepare:

- **Wash all the ingredients thoroughly.**
- **Juice them well and enjoy this fresh drink right away.**

Total calories: 190

Vitamins: Vitamin A 1059ug, Vitamin C 71mg, Calcium 161mg

Minerals: Sodium 192mg, Potassium 1430mg

Sugars 31g

24.   Orange Banana Mix

This is a wonderful juice for people who have serious problems with blood pressure and heart issues. The ingredients in this juice are packed with nutrients that will help strengthen your immune system as well.

Benefits:

Oranges, being high in flavonoids and vitamin C have been known to lower the risk of heart disease. A flavonoid called hesperidin found in oranges can lower high blood pressure.

Ingredients:

- Apples - 2 medium 360g
- Ginger Root - 1/2 thumb 12g
- Lime- ½ 30g
- Orange (peeled) - 1 fruit 130g
- Banana – 1 medium 90g

How to prepare:

- **Wash all the ingredients thoroughly.**

- **Juice them well and enjoy this fresh drink right away.**

Total calories: 166

Vitamins: Vitamin A 15ug, Vitamin C 71mg, Calcium 115mg

Minerals: Sodium 85mg, Potassium 982mg

Sugars 34g

25.   Grapefruit Heart Disease Preventor

This is a great juice to help you prevent blood pressure and heart issues. Grapefruit is a powerful fruit with cholesterol lowering properties. You can add the entire fruit if you don't mind the flavor as it will make it even better for you and your heart.

Benefits:

Including celery in your diet helps protect the body against heart disease and also lowers blood pressure. Carrots have a cleansing effect on the liver and helps it to release more bile.

Ingredients:

- Apple - 1 large 200g
- Grapefruit - 1/2 large peeled 160g
- Beet Root - 1 beet 175g
- Carrots - 4 medium 244g
- Celery - 1 stalk, large 60g

How to prepare:

- **Wash all the ingredients thoroughly.**
- **Juice them well and enjoy this fresh drink right away.**

Total calories: 175

Vitamins: Vitamin A 1632ug, Vitamin C 38mg, Calcium 181mg

Minerals: Sodium 398mg, Potassium 1651mg

Sugars 33g

26. PomePower

Pomegranate is a delicious fruit that will add a distinctive flavor to this juice when added to the other ingredients. Try it morning or afternoon but not recommended for the evening.

Benefits:

Lemon juice helps control high blood pressure and prevents mental stress and depression.

Ingredients:

- Blueberry - 1 cup 145g
- Lemon – 1/2 fruit 30g
- Pomegranate - 1 pomegranate 280g
- Banana – 1 medium 100g

How to prepare:

- **Wash all the ingredients thoroughly.**
- **Juice them well and enjoy this fresh drink right away.**

Total calories: 176

Vitamins: Vitamin A 4ug, Vitamin C 42mg, Calcium 27mg

Minerals: Sodium 6mg, Potassium 580mg

Sugars 35g

27. A Plus Start

What a combination of vitamins and minerals in this juice! Kale and spinach together in one drink is spectacular. Make sure you drink this juice at least once per week.

Benefits:

People who eat two apples per day lower their cholesterol by as much as 15 percent. Apples might also lower blood pressure.

Ingredients:

- Apples - 2 medium 360g
- Kale - 2 leaf 70g
- Spinach - 2 cups 50g
- Lime – ½ fruit 30g

How to prepare:

- **Wash all the ingredients thoroughly.**
- **Juice them well and enjoy this fresh drink right away.**

Total calories: 132

Vitamins: Vitamin A 453ug, Vitamin C 87mg, Calcium 126mg

Minerals: Sodium 51mg, Potassium 815mg

Sugars 25g

28. Carrot Cut

Taste this juice recipe and you will be amazed of how delicious it is, and let's not forget all those vital nutrients that come together. It's a must for people with hypertension.

Benefits:

Pectin in carrots lowers the serum cholesterol levels and some studies show that they might play a role in lowering blood pressure.

Ingredients:

- Apples - 2 medium 360g
- Carrots - 2 medium 120g
- Ginger Root - 1/2 thumb 12g
- Cucumber -1 small 200g

How to prepare:

- **Wash all the ingredients thoroughly.**
- **Juice them well and enjoy this fresh drink right away.**

Total calories: 185

Vitamins: Vitamin A 750ug, Vitamin C 25mg, Calcium 54mg

Minerals: Sodium 48mg, Potassium 609mg

Sugars 27g

29. Peach Adore

It doesn't matter what time of the day it is, this juice recipe can be served at any hour. Check out all the ingredients and get ready for a delicious juice with a truly fantastic flavor.

Benefits:

Peaches might help in maintaining a balanced blood pressure level and also in being a blood purifier.

Ingredients:

- Carrots - 3 medium 130gg
- Lemon - 1/2 fruit 42g
- Peaches - 5 medium 750g
- Orange- 1 medium 120g

How to prepare:

- **Wash all the ingredients thoroughly.**
- **Juice them well and enjoy this fresh drink right away.**

Total calories: 362

Vitamins: Vitamin A 520ug, Vitamin C 71mg, Calcium 215mg

Minerals: Sodium 401mg, Potassium 3024mg

Sugars 7g

30. Sweet P

Here is another great tasting juice with sweet potato that is full of vitamins and minerals. It's very high on beta carotene which is fundamental in preventing hypertension and skin problems.

Benefits:

Sweet potatoes are a good source of nutrients and beets have been shown to help cleanse the blood.

Ingredients:

- Apples - 2 medium 364g
- Beet Root - 1 beet 82g
- Sweet Potato - 1 sweet potato, 130g
- Banana – 1 medium 100g

How to prepare:

- **Wash all the ingredients thoroughly.**
- **Juice them well and enjoy this fresh drink right away.**

Total calories: 201

Vitamins: Vitamin A 640ug, Vitamin C 16mg, Calcium 53mg

Minerals: Sodium 420mg, Potassium 3105mg

Sugars 30g

31. Pineapple Orange Mix

A healthy mind and a healthy body should be the motto of every individual. Add or reduce the amount of ginger root and kale depending on your preference.

Benefits:

Oranges have been shown to help lower blood pressure, and ginger lowers cholesterol.

Ingredients:

- Ginger Root - 1/2 thumb 12g
- Kale - 4 leaf 140g
- Orange - 1 small 96g
- Pineapple - 1 cup, chunks 165g
- Cucumber - 1 300g

How to prepare:

- **Wash all the ingredients thoroughly.**
- **Juice them well and enjoy this fresh drink right away.**

Total calories: 250

Vitamins: Vitamin A 594ug, Vitamin C 241mg, Calcium 203mg

Minerals: Sodium 39mg, Potassium 1160mg

Sugars 40g

32.   Beet Peach Sabore

What's more important than your own health? Take the time to feed your body all the right vitamins and nutrients it needs with this great juice mix. Don't pay attention to the color of the drink as the flavor is what will make the difference.

Benefits:

The high content of iron in beets regenerates and reactivates the red blood cells. They also normalize blood pressure by lowering or elevating it.

Ingredients:

- Apple - 1 medium 180g
- Beet Root - 1 beet 82g
- Lemon - 1/2 fruit 29g
- Peach -1 medium 120g

How to prepare:

- **Wash all the ingredients thoroughly.**

- **Juice them well and enjoy this fresh drink right away.**

Total calories: 180

Vitamins: Vitamin A 10ug, Vitamin C 101mg, Calcium 45mg

Minerals: Sodium 44mg, Potassium 760mg

Sugars 39g

33. Spinach Punch

Juicing has become a very popular way of getting healthy, but is not as popular as it will be in the future. Be a step ahead of everyone by juicing your way to a more controlled blood pressure level with this spinach mix.

Benefits:

Ginger Root is great for lowering blood pressure and reducing the risk of cancer.

Ingredients:

- Apples - 1 medium 180g
- Carrots - 2 medium 120g
- Ginger Root - 1/2 thumb 12g
- Lime - 1 fruit 55g
- Spinach – 2 handful 50g

How to prepare:

- **Wash all the ingredients thoroughly.**
- **Juice them well and enjoy this fresh drink right away.**

Total calories: 193

Vitamins: Vitamin A 1785ug, Vitamin C 98 mg, Calcium 94mg

Minerals: Sodium 156mg, Potassium 1459mg

Sugars 33g

34.   FB Health Mix

Your own health should be treated seriously. Having high blood pressure is serious and should be watched carefully. This juice is a great start towards maintaining your blood pressure stabilized.

Benefits:

Drinking Fennel Bulb juice is helpful for people suffering with heart problems as it contains potassium. Ginger can increase blood circulation and combat fever.

Ingredients:

- Apples - 2 medium 360g
- Fennel Bulb (with fronds) - 1 bulb 230g
- Ginger Root - 1/2 thumb 12g
- Orange (peeled) - 1 fruit 130g

How to prepare:

- **Wash all the ingredients thoroughly.**
- **Juice them well and enjoy this fresh drink right away.**

Total calories: 153

Vitamins: Vitamin A 15ug, Vitamin C 70mg, Calcium 118mg

Minerals: Sodium 79mg, Potassium 1144mg

Sugars 31g

35. Beet Fast

A good solution for any type of health problem is adding fruits and vegetables to your juice recipes. Check out the benefits and all the ingredients you will get from this juice and the different flavor from the parsley.

Benefits:

Parsley has been used in animal studies to help increase the antioxidant capacity of the blood. Beets are useful in helping cleanse the liver, and the liver helps metabolize fat.

Ingredients:

- Apple - 1 medium 180g
- Beet Root - 1/2 beet 40g
- Carrots - 3 medium 180g
- Parsley - 1 handful 40g
- Lime – ½ 30g

How to prepare:

- **Wash all the ingredients thoroughly.**

- **Juice them well and enjoy this fresh drink right away.**

Total calories: 119

Vitamins: Vitamin A 1174ug, Vitamin C 45mg, Calcium 121mg

Minerals: Sodium 190mg, Potassium 1005mg

Sugars 22g

36. Pine A Plus Juice

The combination of pineapple and apple make this juice taste delicious and the other ingredients bring added vitamins that it a great choice to start the day or any time of the day.

Benefits:

Pineapple juice is rich in vitamins and it might help lower blood pressure and even reduce cholesterol levels.

Ingredients:

- Apple - 1 medium 180g
- Lemon - 1/2 fruit 25g
- Orange (peeled) - 1 large 180g
- Pineapple - 1/4 fruit 225g
- Cucumber – 1 300g

How to prepare:

- **Wash all the ingredients thoroughly.**
- **Juice them well and enjoy this fresh drink right away.**

Total calories: 215

Vitamins: Vitamin A 41ug, Vitamin C 140mg, Calcium 90mg

Minerals: Sodium 5mg, Potassium 837mg

Sugars 49g

37. Double Mango Orange

As your body grows older if you don't take care of it, you might encounter different problems. One of them being high blood pressure. This juice recipe will help you to control your hypertension and prevent other future health problems.

Benefits:

Oranges, being high in vitamin C can help stimulate white cells to fight infection, naturally building a good immune system. Mango can help reduce cholesterol.

Ingredients:

- Apple - 1 large 223g
- Lemon (peeled) - 1/2 fruit 29g
- Mango (peeled) - 1 fruit 336g
- Orange - 1 large 184g
- Spinach – 50g

How to prepare:

- **Wash all the ingredients thoroughly.**

- **Juice them well and enjoy this fresh drink right away.**

Total calories: 245

Vitamins: Vitamin A 146ug, Vitamin C 147mg, Calcium 91mg

Minerals: Sodium 4mg, Potassium 860mg

Sugars 50g

38. Orangy Delight

Try this juice recipe and see how the benefits will change the way you feel and perform during the day. You will see after the first day you won't want to miss it another day.

Benefits:

Carrots do wonders for boosting the immune system by increasing the production and performance of white blood cells. Oranges can lower high blood pressure.

Ingredients:

- Apples - 2 large 400g
- Carrots - 5 medium 200g
- Orange - 1 large 184g
- Peaches - 2 large 350g
- Banana – 1 medium 100g

How to prepare:

- **Wash all the ingredients thoroughly.**
- **Juice them well and enjoy this fresh drink right away.**

Total calories: 379

Vitamins: Vitamin A 3376ug, Vitamin C 116mg, Calcium 220mg

Minerals: Sodium 291mg, Potassium 2521mg

Sugars 80g

39. Cranberry Light

This juice recipe is great to server at the end of the day, because it will make your body relax faster before going to bed. It will also supply you with a lot of the vitamins and minerals you will need to start the next day.

Benefits:

Cranberries are a great source of vitamins and minerals. They lower blood pressure and improve blood circulation.

Ingredients:

- Apples - 3 medium 546g
- Cranberries - 1/2 cup, whole 50g
- Ginger Root - 1/4 thumb 6g
- Orange - 1 large (184g
- Lime – ½ fruit 25 g
- Spinach – 50g

How to prepare:

- **Wash all the ingredients thoroughly.**

- **Juice them well and enjoy this fresh drink right away.**

Total calories: 220

Vitamins: Vitamin A 23ug, Vitamin C 87mg, Calcium 80mg

Minerals: Sodium 5mg, Potassium 725mg

Sugars 41g

40. Reduce Stress Mix

If stress is your problem, then you should see what effects this juice recipe will have on you. It's really great and you won't stress about your health as much now that you're getting an overload of nutrients.

Benefits:

Celery calms the nerves because of the high calcium content & helps in controlling high blood pressure. Raw celery should be eaten to reduce high blood pressure.

Ingredients:

- Apple - 1 medium 180g
- Celery - 2 stalk, large 120gg
- Lemon (with peel) - 1/2 fruit 42g
- Banana – 1 medium 100g

How to prepare:

- **Wash all the ingredients thoroughly.**
- **Juice them well and enjoy this fresh drink right away.**

Total calories: 128

Vitamins: Vitamin A 101ug, Vitamin C 87mg, Calcium 140mg

Minerals: Sodium 124mg, Potassium 1027mg

Sugars 19g

41. B Victory

This juice recipe should be on the top of your list. It has a great content of vitamins and minerals. The best time of the day to serve it would be in the morning because it will give you a big energy boost.

Benefits:

Beets are high in carbohydrates, meaning they are a great instant energy source. They are a good blood purifier.

Ingredients:

- Apple - 1 large 200g
- Beet Root - 1 beet 170g
- Carrots - 4 medium 241g
- Celery - 1 stalk, large 60g

How to prepare:

- **Wash all the ingredients thoroughly.**
- **Juice them well and enjoy this fresh drink right away.**

Total calories: 155

Vitamins: Vitamin A 1292ug, Vitamin C 34mg, Calcium 175mg

Minerals: Sodium 300mg, Potassium 1750mg

Sugars 30g

42. Double AA Gulp

After you serve a meal you should wait 30-60 minutes before you can drink this juice recipe. Check the ingredients and how to prepare it before starting. Get ready for a delicious and very healthy source of vitamins and minerals.

Benefits:

Avocados reduce risk of heart disease and help the immune system get stronger.

Ingredients:

- Apples – 1 medium 150g
- Avocado - 1 avocado 188g
- Lime - 1 fruit 60g
- Spinach - 2 cup 60g

How to prepare:

- **Wash all the ingredients thoroughly.**
- **Juice them well and enjoy this fresh drink right away.**

Total calories: 353

Vitamins: Vitamin A 243ug, Vitamin C 47mg, Calcium 164mg

Minerals: Sodium 152mg, Potassium 1788mg

Sugars 20g

43. BALK Juice

If you want to start controlling your hypertension in a fast and effective way, then you should begin with this juice. It's easy to prepare and has a high source of antioxidants necessary to prevent all kinds of diseases.

Benefits:

Several nutrients contained in kiwifruit, including iron, copper and vitamins. Studies indicate that it might help reduce heart disease.

Ingredients:

- Blackberry - 1 cup 120g
- Kiwifruit - 1 fruit 69g
- Apple -2 large 360 g
- Lime – ½ 30 g

How to prepare:

- **Wash all the ingredients thoroughly.**
- **Juice them well and enjoy this fresh drink right away.**

Total calories: 183

Vitamins: Vitamin A 80ug, Vitamin C 110mg, Calcium 75mg

Minerals: Sodium 7mg, Potassium 560mg

Sugars 30g

44. Daily Double Mix

Indeed a healthy lifestyle should consist of doing daily exercises and taking care of your diet. That's why juice recipe should be taken often and in the morning to help you start off your day with a strong dose of beta-carotene.

Benefits:

Celery and apples help lowering high blood pressure, and they are an excellent source of nutrients.

Ingredients:

- 2 large Carrots, 200g
- Tomatoes -1 medium 110g
- Apple – 1 medium 100g
- Celery -1 stalk 50g

How to prepare:

- **Wash all the ingredients thoroughly.**
- **Juice them together and enjoy this fresh drink right away.**

Total calories: 163

Vitamins: Vitamin A 400μg, Vitamin C 15mg, Calcium 20mg

Minerals: Sodium 13mg, Potassium 223 mg

Sugars 15g

45.   Tangy Potato

If you were looking for something that can help blood pressure health problems you should see how this juice recipe is prepared and give it a try. You might want to take it in the morning but can also drink it during the day. It looks great and tastes even better because of all the sweet ingredients it has.

Benefits:

Oranges are a great source of vitamins and may also help in reducing high blood pressure.

Ingredients:

- Apples – 2, 360g
- Celery - 1 stalk, 65g
- Orange (peeled) - 125g
- Sweet Potato - 120g
- Banana – 1 medium 100g

How to prepare:

- **Wash all the ingredients thoroughly.**

- **Juice them together and enjoy this fresh drink right away.**

Total calories: 330

Vitamins: Vitamin A 690µg, Vitamin C 75mg, Calcium 150mg

Minerals: Sodium 76mg, Potassium 349mg

Sugars 55g

46. Power Kick

There are plenty of juice recipes that will bring positive results to your health but this one will is specific for hypertension. You can eliminate the lime if you feel it give it a flavor too strong for your palate.

Benefits:

Carrots increase performance of white blood cells and help eliminate excess fluids from the body. Blood pressure is reduced also by them.

Ingredients:

- Carrots - 2 medium 120g
- Celery - 1 stalk, 50g
- Tomatoes - 2 medium whole 220g
- Banana – 1 medium 100g
- Lime – ½ 25g

How to prepare:

- **Wash all the ingredients thoroughly.**

- **Juice them together and enjoy this fresh drink right away.**

Total calories: 85

Vitamins: Vitamin A 900μg, Vitamin C 140mg, Calcium 197mg

Minerals: Sodium 24mg, Potassium 268mg

Sugars 14g

47. Maximum Strength Mix

This juice recipe is great to serve in the morning because of the strong taste it has and the wonderful effects it will have over your body throughout the day. You can add or reduce the portions to satisfy your needs and to make it to your liking.

Benefits:

Apples are a great source of vitamins and they are also known for lowering high blood pressure and a high content of nutrients.

Ingredients:

- Apples -1 large – 120g
- Ginger Root - 45g
- Grapefruit (peeled)- 300g

How to prepare:

- **Wash all the ingredients thoroughly.**
- **Juice them together and enjoy this fresh drink right away.**

Total calories: 220

Vitamins: Vitamin A 123µg, Vitamin C 200mg, Calcium 139mg

Minerals: Sodium 9mg, Potassium 220mg

Sugars 42g

48. Strawberry Punch Mix

This juice is very high in vitamin C because of all the strawberries that are in it as well as the lemon. The carrots add beta-carotene to the added benefits which makes this an awesome drink.

Benefits:

Strawberries help lower cancer death rates, and are known for lowering the risk of heart disease.

Ingredients:

- Apples – 1 large 120g
- Lemon - 1/2 fruit 32g
- Strawberries - 2 cup, 230g
- Carrot - 1 small, 50g

How to prepare:

- **Wash all the ingredients thoroughly.**
- **Juice them together and enjoy this fresh drink right away.**

Total calories: 190

Vitamins: Vitamin A 11μg, Vitamin C 185mg, Calcium 68mg

Minerals: Sodium 4mg, Potassium 850mg

Sugars 40g

49. Extra Energy Juice

We all know how vegetables and fruits are very healthy for our body that is why you should start drinking juice recipes that contain a large variety of them but with great flavor. This is an unusual drink and can be adapted if you don't like any of the ingredients as it does have a strong flavor.

Benefits:

Studies have shown that Cranberries might lower blood pressure and they are good to boost the immune system.

Ingredients:

- Brussel Sprout – 1 sprout 17g
- Cucumber -1, 300g
- Pineapple – ¼ 220g
- Spinach – 2 handful 50g
- Cranberries – 2 cup 190g

How to prepare:

- **Wash all the ingredients thoroughly.**

- **Juice them together and enjoy this fresh drink right away.**

Total calories: 150

Vitamins: Vitamin A 410μg, Vitamin C 204mg, Calcium 209mg

Minerals: Sodium 79mg, Potassium 470mg

Sugars 34g

50. BOAP Juice

Having time restricted lifestyles and busy days is no excuse for not focusing on controlling your high blood pressure so make sure you do what's necessary to drink your way top better health on a consistent basis.

Benefits:

Oranges being high in vitamin C reduce the risk of heart diseases, and also might lower blood pressure levels.

Ingredients:

- Applet - 1 medium 180g
- Oranges - 2 large 365g
- Peaches - 2 medium 300g
- Banana – 1 medium 120g

How to prepare:

- **Wash all the ingredients thoroughly.**
- **Juice them together and enjoy this fresh drink right away.**

Total of calories: 940

Vitamins: Vitamin A 50μg, Vitamin C 110mg, Calcium 100mg

Minerals: Sodium 30mg, Potassium 120mg

Sugars 40g

OTHER GREAT TITLES BY THIS AUTHOR

Advanced Mental Toughness Training for Bodybuilders

Using Visualization to Push Yourself to the Limit

By

Joseph Correa

Certified Sports Nutritionist

Becoming Mentally Tougher in Bodybuilding by Using Meditation

Reach Your Potential by Controlling Your Inner Thoughts

By

Joseph Correa

Certified Sports Nutritionist

www.ingramcontent.com/pod-product-compliance
Lightning Source LLC
Chambersburg PA
CBHW071721020426
42333CB00017B/2351